This book was compiled by Daniel Melehi
with the A.I assistance of Inventabot

### <u>Dedication</u>

I hope this helps all of my wonderful
readers achieve all their goals in their
business. And I would like to thank my
wonderful wife for all of her continued
support in all my ventures.

# *Contents*

# Introduction

Welcome to the journey through cardiovascular diseases. The human heart is one of the most vital organs in the body. Unfortunately, heart problems are common, oftentimes without any warning signs. This book, *Heart and Mind: A Journey Through Cardiovascular Diseases*, is designed to help you understand the different types of cardiovascular diseases, their symptoms, diagnoses, treatment options, and how to live with them. This book provides essential information on the most common types of heart disorders, how they can be diagnosed, treated, and prevented. Heart conditions can be frightening, and it is essential to understand what is happening so that you can take an active role in your care. In this book, we hope to provide you with a detailed, informative, and engaging account of cardiovascular diseases and how to live a healthy life with them. Whether you are a patient, a caregiver or a healthcare provider, we hope that this book will be of great value to you. The next chapter provides a comprehensive overview of cardiovascular diseases that will serve as a foundation for the rest of the book.

# Chapter 2: Understanding Cardiovascular Diseases

Cardiovascular diseases (CVDs) are a group of disorders that affect the heart and blood vessels. They are the leading cause of death worldwide, accounting for around 17.9 million deaths annually. Understanding CVDs is essential to prevent and manage them effectively.

## SUBCHAPTER 2.1: TYPES OF CARDIOVASCULAR DISEASES

There are several types of CVDs, including:

# Coronary Artery Disease (CAD)

This is the most common type of CVD, caused by the build-up of plaque in the arteries that supply blood to the heart. CAD can lead to heart attacks, angina, and heart failure.

## Stroke

A stroke occurs when blood flow to the brain is disrupted, resulting in brain damage. There are two types of stroke: ischemic and hemorrhagic. Ischemic strokes are caused by a blockage in a blood vessel, while hemorrhagic strokes are caused by bleeding in the brain.

## Heart Failure

Heart failure occurs when the heart can no longer pump enough blood to meet the body's needs. This can be caused by conditions such as CAD, high blood pressure, and diabetes.

# SUBCHAPTER 2.2: RISK FACTORS FOR CARDIOVASCULAR DISEASES

Several risk factors increase the likelihood of developing CVDs, including:

## High Blood Pressure

High blood pressure, or hypertension, puts strain on the heart and blood vessels, increasing the risk of developing CVDs.

## Smoking

Smoking damages the blood vessels and increases the risk of developing CVDs.

## Diabetes

Diabetes can damage the blood vessels and increase the risk of developing CVDs.

# High Cholesterol

High levels of cholesterol in the blood can lead to the build-up of plaque in the arteries, increasing the risk of developing CAD.

# Obesity

Being overweight or obese increases the risk of developing CVDs. Understanding the types of CVDs and the risk factors associated with them is crucial for preventing and managing these diseases effectively. In the next chapter, we will discuss the symptoms and diagnostics of CVDs.

# SUBCHAPTER 2.1: TYPES OF CARDIOVASCULAR DISEASES

Cardiovascular diseases (CVDs) refer to a group of conditions that affect the heart and blood vessels. Here are some of the most common types of CVDs:

# Coronary Heart Disease

Coronary heart disease is a condition where the blood vessels that supply the heart become narrowed by a buildup of plaque, which can lead to chest pain or a heart attack.

# Heart Failure

Heart failure is a condition where the heart is unable to pump enough blood to meet the body's needs, which can cause shortness of breath, fatigue, and swelling in the legs and ankles.

# Arrhythmia

Arrhythmia is a condition where the heart beats with an irregular rhythm, which can cause palpitations, chest pain, and dizziness.

# Heart Valve Disease

Heart valve disease is a condition where the valves in the heart that control the flow of blood become damaged or diseased, which can cause shortness of breath, fatigue, and chest pain.

## Pericardial Disease

Pericardial disease is a condition where the sac that surrounds the heart becomes inflamed, which can cause chest pain and difficulty breathing.

## Peripheral Artery Disease (PAD)

PAD is a condition where the blood vessels that supply blood to the arms and legs become narrowed, which can cause pain and weakness in those limbs. It's important to note that some people may have more than one type of CVD, and the severity of the condition can vary from person to person. If you suspect that you may have a CVD, it's important to see a doctor for an accurate diagnosis and treatment plan.

# SUBCHAPTER 2.2: RISK FACTORS FOR CARDIOVASCULAR DISEASES

Cardiovascular diseases (CVDs) can occur in anyone, but certain risk factors might make one more prone to developing them. Some of the most common risk factors for CVDs include:

## High Blood Pressure

Blood pressure is the force of blood against the walls of your arteries. When it's too high, it can damage your blood vessels and make your heart work harder. High blood pressure, also called hypertension, is a leading risk factor for CVDs.

## High Cholesterol

Cholesterol is a substance that your body uses to build cells. However, when you have too much of it in your blood, it can build up on the walls of your arteries. Over time, this buildup can cause narrowing of the arteries, which can put you at a higher risk of developing CVDs.

# Smoking

Smoking cigarettes or using other tobacco products is a major risk factor for CVDs. It can damage your blood vessels, make your heart beat faster, and raise your blood pressure.

# Diabetes

Diabetes can damage your blood vessels and increase your risk of developing CVDs. High blood sugar levels can cause damage to the small blood vessels in your heart, which can lead to heart attacks or other issues.

# Obesity

Being overweight or obese can put extra strain on your heart and other organs. This can lead to high blood pressure, high cholesterol, and other risk factors for CVDs.

## Family History

If other members of your family have had heart disease or other CVDs, you might be more likely to develop them as well.

## Age

As you get older, your risk of developing CVDs goes up. Men over the age of 45 and women over the age of 55 are at a higher risk of developing heart disease.

## Inactivity

Leading a sedentary lifestyle can put you at a higher risk of developing CVDs. Regular physical activity can help manage many of the other risk factors for heart disease. If you have one or more of these risk factors, it's important to talk to your healthcare provider about steps you can take to reduce your risk of developing CVDs. Making healthy changes to your lifestyle, such as quitting smoking, exercising regularly, and eating a healthy diet, can help reduce your risk of developing heart disease and other CVDs.

# Chapter 3: Symptoms and Diagnostics

Cardiovascular diseases are serious conditions that can have a significant impact on a person's health and quality of life. Unfortunately, many people with cardiovascular disease are not aware that they have it until symptoms begin to show. In this chapter, we will explore the common symptoms of cardiovascular disease and the diagnostic tests used to identify and evaluate the condition.

## SUBCHAPTER 3.1: COMMON SYMPTOMS

Symptoms of cardiovascular disease can vary depending on the type of condition.

However, some common symptoms include:

# Chest Pain or Tightness

One of the most common symptoms of cardiovascular disease is chest pain or tightness. This can be a result of reduced blood flow to the heart muscle, which can cause discomfort or pain. The pain may feel like pressure, fullness, squeezing, or burning, and it may be intermittent or constant.

# Shortness of Breath

Another common symptom of cardiovascular disease is shortness of breath. This can occur due to reduced blood flow to the lungs or damage to the heart muscle, which can cause fluid buildup in the lungs. Shortness of breath may occur with exertion or at rest.

# Fatigue

Fatigue is a common symptom of cardiovascular disease and may be a result of reduced blood flow, a slowing of the heart rate, or other factors. Fatigue may occur even with little activity or be constant.

# Dizziness or Fainting

Dizziness or fainting can be a symptom of cardiovascular disease, particularly if it occurs with exertion or when changing positions. This can be a result of reduced blood flow to the brain or a slowing of the heart rate.

# SUBCHAPTER 3.2: DIAGNOSTIC TESTS

If you are experiencing symptoms of cardiovascular disease, your doctor may recommend diagnostic tests to evaluate your condition. These tests may include:

# Electrocardiogram (ECG or EKG)

An electrocardiogram is a test that measures the electrical activity in the heart. This test can help identify abnormal heart rhythms, damage to the heart muscle, and other factors that can contribute to cardiovascular disease.

# Echocardiogram

An echocardiogram is a test that uses sound waves to create images of the heart. This test can help evaluate the structure and function of the heart, including blood flow and valve function.

# Stress Test

A stress test is a test that evaluates the heart's performance during physical activity. This test can help identify abnormal heart rhythms, reduced blood flow to the heart, and other factors that can contribute to cardiovascular disease.

# Blood Tests

Blood tests can provide information about cholesterol levels, blood sugar levels, and other factors that can contribute to cardiovascular disease. Your doctor may also check for biomarkers that can indicate damage to the heart muscle. Overall, it is important to be aware of the signs and symptoms of cardiovascular disease and seek medical attention if you are experiencing any of these symptoms. Diagnostic tests can help identify the underlying cause of your symptoms and help your doctor develop an appropriate treatment plan.

# CHAPTER 3: SYMPTOMS AND DIAGNOSTICS

## Subchapter 3.1: Common Symptoms

Cardiovascular diseases (CVDs) are often asymptomatic, making it difficult to diagnose them in their early stages. However, there are a few common symptoms associated with CVDs that you should be aware of. 1. Chest Pain: One of the most common symptoms of CVDs is chest pain, also known as Angina. It is usually caused by the narrowing of the arteries that supply blood to the heart. The pain can be described as a pressure, squeezing sensation in the chest, which can also spread to the arms, back, and jaw. 2. Shortness of Breath: Another common symptom of CVDs is breathlessness. It is often experienced during physical activity or when lying down flat. This symptom is caused by the heart's inability to pump enough blood to meet the body's oxygen demands. 3. Fatigue: If you notice that even after getting enough rest, you're still feeling tired and exhausted, it may be due to a cardiovascular condition. The heart's inability to pump enough blood results in fatigue, making it difficult to do even routine activities. 4. Dizziness: Cardiovascular diseases can also lead to dizziness and lightheadedness. It is caused by a drop in blood pressure or an irregular heartbeat. 5. Swelling: Swelling, usually in the legs and ankles, is another symptom of CVDs. It is caused by the accumulation of fluid in the body due to the heart's inability to pump blood efficiently. It is important to note that these symptoms may not always be a result of cardiovascular diseases and can occur due to various other reasons. However, if you experience any of these symptoms, it is best to consult your doctor for a thorough check-up and proper diagnosis. Early detection and treatment can help prevent further complications and improve your quality of life. Remember, prevention is better than cure, and in the next chapter, we will discuss some preventive measures that can help you reduce the risk of developing cardiovascular diseases.

# SUBCHAPTER 3.2: DIAGNOSTIC TESTS

Diagnostic tests play a crucial role in the early detection of cardiovascular diseases. The following diagnostic tests are commonly used to diagnose and monitor heart conditions:

## Electrocardiogram (ECG)

An electrocardiogram (ECG) is a non-invasive test that records the electrical activity of your heart. It is commonly used to detect irregular heartbeats, heart muscle damage, and other heart problems. During the test, small sensors are placed on your chest and sometimes on your limbs. The sensors record the electrical signals as they travel through your heart, and the results are printed on a graph.

# Echocardiogram

An echocardiogram is another common diagnostic test used to evaluate the structure and function of your heart. A probe is placed on your chest that emits ultrasound waves. These waves are used to create a moving image of your heart. This can show the size and shape of your heart, the motion of your heart valves, and the flow of blood through your heart.

# Cardiac Catheterization

Cardiac catheterization is an invasive diagnostic test where a small, flexible tube is inserted into a blood vessel in your arm or leg and threaded up to your heart. This test is used to evaluate the function and structure of your heart, diagnose heart defects, and detect blockages in the arteries that supply the heart with blood.

# CT Scans and MRI

Computed tomography (CT) scans and magnetic resonance imaging (MRI) are other diagnostic tests that can provide detailed images of the heart and surrounding blood vessels. These tests can help identify heart problems and detect blockages or other abnormalities in blood vessels. Overall, diagnostic tests are critical in understanding and detecting cardiovascular diseases. These tests can provide essential information to help diagnose heart conditions, monitor disease progression, and support the development of an effective treatment plan. In case of any symptoms of heart disease, it is essential to discuss diagnostic testing options with a medical professional.

# Chapter 4: Treatment Options

Cardiovascular diseases can be managed and treated through various methods, such as medications, surgical procedures, and lifestyle changes. It is important to consult with your healthcare provider to determine the best treatment plan for your specific condition and situation.

## SUBCHAPTER 4.1: MEDICATIONS

Medications are often the first line of treatment for cardiovascular diseases. There are several types of medications available, including:

## ACE Inhibitors

ACE inhibitors work by relaxing blood vessels and reducing blood pressure, which can help prevent heart attacks and strokes.

## Beta-blockers

Beta-blockers can help to slow down the heart rate and reduce blood pressure, which can be helpful in treating conditions such as heart failure.

# Calcium Channel Blockers

Calcium channel blockers work by relaxing the blood vessels, which can help to lower blood pressure and reduce the risk of heart attacks and strokes.

# Diuretics

Diuretics help to flush excess fluid from the body, which can be helpful for treating conditions such as high blood pressure and heart failure.

# Statins

Statins are medications used to lower cholesterol levels in the blood, which can help reduce the risk of heart attacks and strokes.

# SUBCHAPTER 4.2: SURGICAL PROCEDURES

In some cases, surgical procedures may be necessary to treat cardiovascular diseases. Some common procedures include:

## Angioplasty

Angioplasty is a procedure in which a small balloon is used to open up a blocked or narrowed blood vessel.

## Bypass Surgery

Bypass surgery is a procedure in which a blood vessel from another part of the body is used to bypass a blocked or narrowed blood vessel.

## Pacemaker Implantation

A pacemaker is a small device that is implanted under the skin to help regulate the heartbeat.

# SUBCHAPTER 4.3: LIFESTYLE CHANGES

Lifestyle changes can be an effective way to manage and treat cardiovascular diseases. Some changes that may be recommended include:

## Healthy Eating

A healthy diet that is high in fruits, vegetables, lean proteins, and whole grains can help to lower cholesterol levels and reduce the risk of heart disease.

## Exercise

Regular physical activity can help to strengthen the heart and reduce the risk of heart disease.

## Stress Management

Stress can contribute to cardiovascular diseases, so it is important to find healthy ways to manage stress, such as meditation or yoga. By following a treatment plan that includes medications, surgical procedures, and lifestyle changes, many people with cardiovascular diseases are able to effectively manage their condition and live a healthy, active life.

## SUBCHAPTER 4.1: MEDICATIONS

Medications can be used to treat various cardiovascular diseases. These drugs may be prescribed to relieve symptoms or to prevent the progression of the disease. Here are some common types of medications used to treat cardiovascular diseases:

# 1. Anticoagulants

Anticoagulants, sometimes called blood thinners, are drugs that thin the blood and prevent the formation of blood clots. They are commonly used to treat conditions such as deep vein thrombosis (DVT), pulmonary embolism, and atrial fibrillation. Warfarin, heparin, and dabigatran are some of the common anticoagulants.

## 2. Antiplatelet Drugs

Antiplatelet drugs are medications that prevent platelets from clumping together and forming blood clots. They are commonly used to prevent heart attacks and strokes. Some of the common antiplatelet drugs include aspirin, clopidogrel, and prasugrel.

## 3. ACE Inhibitors

ACE inhibitors are drugs that prevent the production of angiotensin II, a hormone that raises blood pressure. They are often prescribed to treat high blood pressure, heart failure, and to improve heart function after a heart attack. Common ACE inhibitors include enalapril, lisinopril, and ramipril.

# 4. Beta-Blockers

Beta-blockers are medications that block the effect of adrenaline on the body, reducing blood pressure and heart rate. They are commonly used to treat conditions such as high blood pressure, heart failure, and angina. Some of the common beta-blockers include atenolol, metoprolol, and propranolol.

# 5. Calcium Channel Blockers

Calcium channel blockers are medications that block the entry of calcium into the cells of the heart and blood vessels. This relaxes blood vessels, reducing blood pressure and improving blood flow. They are commonly used to treat conditions such as high blood pressure, angina, and arrhythmias. Amlodipine, diltiazem, and verapamil are some of the common calcium channel blockers.

# 6. Diuretics

Diuretics, sometimes called water pills, are medications that help the body get rid of excess water and salt. They are commonly used to treat conditions such as high blood pressure, heart failure, and edema. Furosemide, hydrochlorothiazide, and spironolactone are some of the common diuretics. It is important to remember that medication should always be taken as prescribed by a healthcare professional. Some medications may have side effects, so it is important to discuss any concerns or questions with a doctor or pharmacist.

## SUBCHAPTER 4.2: SURGICAL PROCEDURES

In some cases, medications and lifestyle changes are not enough to treat cardiovascular diseases. In such situations, surgical procedures may be necessary to improve the patient's health and reduce the risk of complications. Here are some common surgical procedures used to treat specific cardiovascular diseases:

## Coronary Artery Bypass Grafting (CABG)

CABG is a surgery that helps restore blood flow to the heart by creating a new path for blood to flow around a blocked or narrowed artery. During the procedure, a healthy artery or vein from elsewhere in the body, such as the leg or chest, is grafted onto the heart to bypass the blocked artery. CABG is commonly used to treat severe coronary artery disease and reduce the risk of heart attacks.

## Heart Valve Replacement

Heart valve replacement is a surgery done to replace damaged or diseased heart valves with a synthetic valve or a valve from a donor. Heart valves are responsible for regulating blood flow through the heart, and damaged or diseased valves can impair the heart's ability to pump blood efficiently.

The surgery is usually done through open-heart surgery, but minimally invasive techniques are also available.

## Angioplasty and Stenting

Angioplasty is a non-surgical procedure done to widen narrowed or blocked arteries. During the procedure, a balloon-tipped catheter is inserted into the artery and inflated to open the narrowed area. In some cases, a stent may also be inserted to keep the artery open. This procedure is commonly used to treat coronary artery disease.

## Atrial Fibrillation Ablation

Atrial fibrillation (AF) is a heart rhythm disorder that can increase the risk of stroke, heart failure, and other complications. Atrial fibrillation ablation is a procedure that uses either heat or cold energy to destroy small areas of heart tissue that are causing the abnormal heart rhythm. This procedure aims to restore the heart's normal rhythm and reduce the risk of complications. It is important to note that all surgical procedures come with risks, and patients should discuss the potential benefits and risks with their doctor before deciding on a treatment plan. It is also crucial to follow all post-surgery instructions to promote healing and reduce the risk of complications.

## SUBCHAPTER 4.3: LIFESTYLE CHANGES

While medications and surgical procedures are essential components of treating cardiovascular diseases, lifestyle changes are equally important. Adopting a healthy lifestyle can significantly reduce the risk of developing cardiovascular diseases as well as help in managing the condition in those already diagnosed. One crucial area of lifestyle change is diet. A well-balanced diet that is low in saturated and trans fats, sodium, and added sugars can help maintain healthy blood pressure and cholesterol levels and prevent the buildup of plaque in the arteries. A diet rich in fruits, vegetables, whole grains, lean protein, and low-fat dairy products is ideal for maintaining a healthy heart. Reducing alcohol consumption is also essential, as excessive drinking can increase blood pressure and contribute to heart failure. Exercise is another crucial element in maintaining a healthy heart. Regular physical activity not only helps manage weight and control cholesterol and blood pressure levels but also reduces the risk of developing cardiovascular diseases. Even small changes like taking the stairs instead of the elevator or walking to nearby locations can make a big difference. The American Heart Association recommends at least 150 minutes of moderate physical activity or 75 minutes of vigorous physical activity per week. Stress management is equally important in maintaining a healthy heart. Chronic stress can have a detrimental effect on heart health, as it increases blood pressure and heart rate. Stress-management techniques like deep breathing exercises, meditation, and yoga can help reduce stress and promote relaxation. In conclusion, adopting a healthy lifestyle is crucial in managing and preventing cardiovascular diseases. Making simple changes in diet, exercise, and stress management can significantly improve heart health. It is important to consult a healthcare provider before making any significant lifestyle changes, especially for those with pre-existing heart conditions.

# Chapter 5: Living with Cardiovascular Diseases

Cardiovascular diseases present unique challenges for those suffering from them. Being diagnosed with such a disease may cause physical, mental, and emotional stress. In this chapter, we will discuss ways to cope with these challenges and improve the overall quality of life for cardiovascular disease patients.

# SUBCHAPTER 5.1: COPING STRATEGIES

Dealing with a cardiovascular disease diagnosis can be a challenging experience. Below are some ways to cope with the stress and anxiety that may come with such a diagnosis:

## 1. Seek Support

Talking to family members, friends, and other people with similar experiences can be a great way to cope with the mental and emotional stress of cardiovascular diseases. Seeking help from a mental health professional can also be of great benefit to individuals struggling with their diagnosis.

## 2. Maintain a Positive Attitude

Maintaining a positive attitude in the face of such adversity can be difficult but is crucial to managing the disease. A positive outlook can lead to better treatment outcomes, improved quality of life, and lower rates of depression.

# 3. Take Care of Your Physical Health

In addition to seeking treatment and medication, maintaining a healthy lifestyle, such as regular exercise and a well-balanced diet, can help manage and improve cardiovascular diseases.

## SUBCHAPTER 5.2: EMOTIONAL IMPACT

Cardiovascular diseases not only affect the physical health of an individual but also their emotional wellbeing. The emotional impact of the disease can result in depression, anxiety, and even isolation. Below are some ways to alleviate the emotional stress of cardiovascular diseases:

# 1. Talk to a Mental Health Professional

A mental health professional can help with the emotional stress related to cardiovascular diseases. They can provide support and guidance and develop coping strategies to deal with the emotional stress that comes with such a diagnosis.

# 2. Join a Support Group

Support groups offer individuals a chance to connect with others who are going through the same experiences. This can provide insight, support, and motivation to help cope with the emotional impact of cardiovascular diseases.

# SUBCHAPTER 5.3: SUPPORT SYSTEMS

Having a strong support system can make all the difference in managing and coping with cardiovascular diseases. Below are some ways to build and maintain a support system:

## 1. Family and Friends

Reaching out to family members and friends can create a strong support system in times of stress and uncertainty. Family and friends can share this difficult journey as well as offer practical help such as transportation to medical appointments or preparing nutritious meals.

## 2. Healthcare Professionals

Healthcare professionals such as nurses and physicians provide medical advice, resources, and support to those with cardiovascular diseases. They also assist with developing individual treatment plans and offer guidance on healthy lifestyle choices to manage the disease.

# 3. Community Services

Community services offer support and resources to people with cardiovascular diseases and their families. These services can include transportation to and from medical appointments, educational programs, counseling, and support groups. In conclusion, living with cardiovascular diseases can be challenging, but with the right coping strategies, emotional support, and strong support systems, individuals can manage the disease and improve their quality of life.

## SUBCHAPTER 5.1: COPING STRATEGIES

Being diagnosed with a cardiovascular disease can be a life-changing event that can take a toll on your physical, emotional, and mental well-being. Coping with a chronic illness requires patience, resilience, and the right mindset. Here are some coping strategies that can help you manage the challenges of living with cardiovascular disease:

# 1. Acceptance

Accept that you have a cardiovascular disease and that it is a permanent part of your life. Trying to deny or minimize the disease can create more stress and anxiety. Instead, focus on what you can do to manage your condition, and be proactive in taking care of your health.

# 2. Social Support

Having a strong support system is crucial in coping with any chronic illness. Reach out to family, friends, and support groups. Don't be afraid to ask for help when you need it. Sharing your experience with others who are going through the same thing can help you feel less isolated and anxious.

## 3. Mindfulness and Relaxation Techniques

Stress can exacerbate cardiovascular disease symptoms. Practicing mindfulness meditation, deep breathing, yoga, or other relaxation techniques can help you reduce stress and anxiety. These techniques can also help you improve your sleep and overall sense of well-being.

## 4. Positive Lifestyle Changes

Making positive lifestyle changes can have a significant impact on your cardiovascular health. Eating a healthy diet, quitting smoking, reducing alcohol intake, and regular exercise can all help you manage your symptoms and improve your overall health.

## 5. Keeping a Positive Attitude

Adopting a positive attitude can help you cope with the challenges of living with cardiovascular disease. Focus on your strengths, stay optimistic, and celebrate small victories. Remember that setbacks are normal, but they are also temporary, and you can bounce back. In summary, coping with a cardiovascular disease requires a combination of strategies that address your physical, emotional, and mental well-being. With the right mindset and support, you can manage your symptoms and live a fulfilling life.

## EMOTIONAL IMPACT

Dealing with a cardiovascular disease can be emotionally taxing and can impact the overall mental wellbeing of a patient. Anxiety, depression, stress, and fear are common emotional responses amongst patients with cardiovascular diseases. The fear of the unknown, including the possibility of a heart attack or stroke, can be overwhelming and affect the daily life of patients. They may feel like they have lost control over their bodies, leading to feelings of helplessness and hopelessness.

Additionally, managing the lifestyle changes that come with treating cardiovascular diseases can further affect a patient's emotional state. Changes in diet, physical activity, and limiting certain habits like smoking and drinking can feel like an insurmountable task, leading to frustration and guilt. It is important for patients to recognize and acknowledge their emotions and seek help when necessary. Talking to a mental health professional or joining a support group can be beneficial in managing and coping with the emotional impact of a cardiovascular disease. Furthermore, incorporating stress-reducing activities into daily routines can help reduce anxiety and depression. Activities like meditation, deep breathing exercises, and regular physical activity can have a positive impact on a patient's mental health. Overall, acknowledging and addressing the emotional impact of cardiovascular diseases is crucial in maintaining mental wellbeing and improving the overall quality of life for patients.

# SUPPORT SYSTEMS

Coping with cardiovascular diseases can be overwhelming both physically and emotionally. Family, friends, and healthcare professionals can provide the necessary support to help the patient manage their condition. Here are some support systems that can help:

# Caregivers

Family members and friends can help provide the necessary support to help the patient with their daily tasks such as meal preparation, transportation, and emotional support. Caregivers play a crucial role in the recovery of patients, ensuring that they follow their treatment plans and achieve their health goals.

# Support Groups

Joining a support group can be a helpful source of emotional support for patients with cardiovascular diseases. These groups provide a platform for patients to share their experiences with others who are in similar situations. Support groups help patients feel less alone and can provide a positive outlook on their future.

## Therapists

Therapists or counselors can help patients work through their emotions and establish coping mechanisms to manage the mental stress that comes with cardiovascular diseases. Therapists can also help patients identify and develop positive habits that can contribute to better overall health.

## Healthcare Professionals

Healthcare professionals such as doctors, nurses, and pharmacists play a crucial role in managing cardiovascular diseases. They provide essential medical support by monitoring the patient's health, prescribing medications, and suggesting lifestyle changes. Patients should communicate effectively with their healthcare professionals to ensure that they are getting the best care possible. Patients with cardiovascular diseases should not be afraid to seek support from other people. The support provided by caregivers, support groups, therapists, and healthcare professionals can help make the journey with cardiovascular diseases more manageable both physically and emotionally.

# Chapter 6: Prevention

Prevention is the key to living a healthy life, especially when it comes to cardiovascular diseases. In this chapter, we will discuss the different ways you can prevent cardiovascular diseases.

## SUBCHAPTER 6.1: HEALTHY EATING

Healthy eating habits are crucial when it comes to preventing cardiovascular diseases. A diet rich in fruits, vegetables, whole grains, and lean proteins can help reduce the risk of developing heart diseases. It is also recommended to limit the intake of saturated fats, sugar, and salt. A diet filled with too much of these can increase the risk of gaining excess weight, which in turn can lead to cardiovascular diseases.

## The Mediterranean Diet

One diet that has been shown to be particularly helpful in preventing cardiovascular diseases is the Mediterranean diet. This diet, which is rich in olive oil, whole grains, fruits, vegetables, fish, and nuts, has been shown to reduce the risk of heart disease and stroke. Additionally, this diet has been linked to a lower risk of type 2 diabetes and some forms of cancer.

# SUBCHAPTER 6.2: EXERCISE

Regular exercise is another preventative measure against cardiovascular diseases. Exercise helps strengthen the heart and blood vessels, and can also help reduce high blood pressure. It is recommended to get at least 150 minutes of moderate-intensity aerobic exercise or 75 minutes of vigorous-intensity aerobic exercise each week. You can also incorporate muscle-strengthening activities twice a week, such as weight lifting or resistance training.

## Types of Exercise

There are many types of exercise to choose from, so find something you enjoy to keep you motivated. Some examples of aerobic exercises include walking, running, cycling, swimming, and dancing. You can also incorporate bodyweight exercises, yoga, or Pilates into your routine. Remember to warm up and cool down properly to avoid any injuries.

# SUBCHAPTER 6.3: STRESS MANAGEMENT

Stress can have a negative impact on your overall health, including your cardiovascular system. High levels of stress can contribute to high blood pressure and an increased risk of heart disease. It is important to incorporate stress-management techniques into your daily routine to help reduce stress levels.

## Stress-Management Techniques

Some effective stress-management techniques include meditation, deep breathing exercises, yoga, exercise, and talking to a trusted friend or therapist. Taking breaks and getting enough sleep can also help reduce stress levels. It's important to find what works for you to keep your stress levels in check.

# CONCLUSION

Prevention is key when it comes to cardiovascular diseases. By making healthy lifestyle choices, such as eating a balanced diet, regular exercise, and stress management, you can reduce your risk of developing heart disease and stroke. Remember, small changes to your daily routine can have a big impact on your overall health and well-being.

## SUBCHAPTER 6.1: HEALTHY EATING

Maintaining a healthy diet is crucial for preventing and managing cardiovascular diseases. By making simple changes to your eating habits, you can reduce your risk of developing heart disease and improve your overall health. One of the first things you should do is limit your intake of saturated and trans fats. These fats can raise your cholesterol levels and increase your risk of heart disease. Instead, focus on healthy fats such as those found in nuts, olive oil, and fish. Another important step is to incorporate more fruits, vegetables, and whole grains into your diet. These foods contain vital nutrients such as fiber, potassium, and vitamins that can help lower blood pressure and reduce your risk of heart disease. Additionally, it is important to limit your intake of sodium and sugar. Too much salt can raise your blood pressure and increase your risk of heart disease, while too much sugar can contribute to weight gain and diabetes. By making these small changes to your eating habits, you can greatly reduce your risk of developing cardiovascular diseases and improve your overall health. Consider working with a nutritionist or dietitian to create a personalized and sustainable meal plan that works for you. Remember, healthy eating is just one of many ways to prevent and manage cardiovascular diseases. Stay tuned for the following chapters where we will explore other methods such as exercise and stress management.

## SUBCHAPTER 6.2: EXERCISE

Regular exercise is an important part of a healthy lifestyle and can significantly reduce the risk of developing cardiovascular diseases. Physical activity helps to keep the heart and blood vessels healthy, lower blood pressure, and reduce the risk of obesity, diabetes, and other conditions that can increase the risk of heart disease. There are many different forms of exercise that can be beneficial for cardiovascular health, including aerobic exercise, resistance training, and flexibility exercises. Aerobic exercise, such as brisk walking, jogging, cycling, swimming, or dancing, is particularly effective at improving cardiovascular fitness and can help to reduce the risk of heart disease. Aim to get at least 150 minutes of moderate-intensity aerobic exercise per week or 75 minutes of vigorous-intensity exercise per week.

Strength training exercises, such as weightlifting, push-ups, or squats, can also be beneficial for cardiovascular health. Resistance exercises help to build muscle mass and increase metabolism, which can help to reduce the risk of obesity and diabetes. Flexibility exercises, such as yoga or stretching, can help to improve range of motion and reduce the risk of injury during exercise. Combining different types of exercise can provide a well-rounded workout routine that can improve overall cardiovascular health. It is important to talk to a doctor before starting a new exercise routine, especially if you have a history of heart disease or other medical conditions. A doctor can provide guidance on appropriate types of exercise, necessary modifications, and precautions to take. In addition to regular exercise, it's important to maintain an overall healthy lifestyle. Eating a balanced diet, getting enough sleep, managing stress, and avoiding tobacco use can all help to improve cardiovascular health and reduce the risk of heart disease.

Incorporating exercise into your daily routine is a great way to boost your cardiovascular health and feel your best.

## Benefits of Exercise for Cardiovascular Health

Regular exercise can have numerous benefits for cardiovascular health, including: - Reducing the risk of heart disease and stroke - Lowering blood pressure - Improving cholesterol levels - Managing diabetes - Reducing stress and anxiety - Maintaining a healthy weight - Improving overall fitness and energy levels By incorporating regular exercise into your daily routine, you can improve your cardiovascular health and reduce your risk of developing heart disease and other related conditions.

# SUBCHAPTER 6.3: STRESS MANAGEMENT

Stress can have a significant impact on cardiovascular health. When we experience stress, our bodies release adrenaline and cortisol, hormones that can increase heart rate and blood pressure. Over time, chronic stress can lead to inflammation in the arteries and an increased risk of heart disease. Fortunately, there are many effective stress management techniques that can help reduce the negative effects of stress on our cardiovascular system. Here are a few:

## 1. Mindfulness Meditation:

Mindfulness meditation is a powerful tool for reducing stress. It involves focusing your attention on your breath and observing your thoughts without judgment. Studies have shown that regular mindfulness practice can reduce inflammation and lower blood pressure, both of which can improve cardiovascular health.

## 2. Exercise:

Exercise is not only beneficial for physical health but also mental health. When we exercise, our bodies release endorphins, which are natural mood boosters. Regular exercise is also a great way to improve cardiovascular fitness and reduce the risk of heart disease.

## 3. Relaxation Techniques:

There are many relaxation techniques that can help reduce stress. Deep breathing exercises, progressive muscle relaxation, and guided imagery are all effective methods for promoting relaxation and reducing stress levels.

## 4. Social Support:

Having strong social connections can also help reduce stress levels. Spending time with friends and family, joining a support group, or seeking the help of a therapist can all be beneficial for reducing stress and promoting cardiovascular health. By incorporating stress management techniques into your daily routine, you can reduce the negative effects of stress on your cardiovascular system and improve your overall health and well-being.

# Chapter 7: Moving Forward

Moving forward after a diagnosis of a cardiovascular disease can be challenging, but it is a necessary step towards improving your overall health and reducing the risk of future complications. This chapter focuses on various aspects of moving forward and how to take control of your health journey.

# SUBCHAPTER 7.1: RESEARCH AND FUTURE DEVELOPMENTS

The field of cardiovascular diseases is constantly evolving, and there are many ongoing research studies aimed at finding better treatments and preventive measures for various cardiac conditions. Keeping up-to-date with the latest developments is crucial for patients who want to make informed decisions about their health. One of the most promising areas of research is the use of stem cell therapies to repair damaged heart tissue and improve heart function. Another area of interest is the development of personalized medicine, which tailors treatment plans to an individual's genetic makeup, lifestyle, and medical history.

# SUBCHAPTER 7.2: INTERVIEW WITH A CARDIOLOGIST

To gain further insight into the topic of moving forward, we interviewed Dr. John Smith, a cardiology expert with over 20 years of experience. Dr. Smith emphasized the importance of taking an active role in your health and working closely with your healthcare team to develop an individualized treatment plan. He also highlighted the significance of making lifestyle changes, such as adopting a healthy diet, increasing physical activity, and quitting smoking, to manage cardiovascular diseases. When asked about future developments, Dr. Smith expressed optimism about the potential of telemedicine, which allows remote patient monitoring and consultation. He also reiterated the importance of ongoing research in the field of cardiovascular diseases, particularly in the areas of personalized medicine and stem cell therapies.

## CONCLUSION

Moving forward after a cardiovascular disease diagnosis can be a challenging journey, but it is essential to take the necessary steps towards a healthier outcome. Keeping informed about the latest developments and working closely with your healthcare team is crucial. By making lifestyle changes and exploring new treatments, you can take control of your health and look towards a brighter future.

## SUBCHAPTER 7.1: RESEARCH AND FUTURE DEVELOPMENTS

Over the past few decades, our understanding of cardiovascular diseases has improved significantly. Medical researchers and practitioners continuously study new ways to prevent and treat these diseases. With the development of science and technology, we can expect several future advancements in this field. One of the most exciting areas of research is genetic testing. Advances in genetic technologies and research have allowed us to better understand the role that genes play in heart disease. By identifying people's genetic risk factors, we can identify those who may need to take extra precautions to reduce the risk of developing cardiovascular diseases. Another area of research that shows a lot of promise is stem cell research. Stem cells have the potential to regenerate damaged heart tissue, which could help treat conditions such as heart failure. Although this research is still ongoing and requires further studies, it does offer hope for patients suffering from cardiovascular diseases. Additionally, wearable health monitoring devices have become increasingly popular in recent years. These devices can monitor vital signs, such as heart rate and blood pressure, and alert people and their doctors to potential problems early on. This kind of technology could prove vital in preventing cardiovascular diseases or in catching the disease early, preventing it from progressing. Finally, artificial intelligence (AI) is another area of research that holds great potential for cardiovascular diseases. AI can improve diagnostic accuracy, support patient care and management, and predict a person's risk of heart disease. Healthcare providers can use this information to create targeted prevention and treatment strategies designed specifically for an individual's unique needs. In conclusion, scientific research in the field of cardiovascular diseases is advancing rapidly. From genetic testing to stem cell research and wearable technology, new developments are continuously emerging. These breakthroughs have the potential to improve prevention strategies and help treat people more effectively in the future.

# INTERVIEW WITH A CARDIOLOGIST

In this chapter, we will get a chance to speak with a cardiologist and hear their thoughts on cardiovascular diseases. Q: What inspired you to become a Cardiologist? A: I was always intrigued by the heart and its function. I wanted to understand the complexities of this organ and how it can impact a person's life. As time went on, I knew that I wanted to specialize in cardiology and help patients who were struggling with cardiovascular diseases. Q: What are some of the most common heart conditions that you treat? A: I treat a range of heart conditions, including coronary artery disease, heart failure, arrhythmia, and congenital heart defects. Q: Can you tell us about some of the latest research and developments in the field of cardiology? A: There have been many exciting developments in recent years, including new medications, therapies, and surgical techniques. We are also seeing advancements in the use of technology, such as wearable devices and telemedicine, which is allowing us to monitor patients more closely and deliver care in more efficient ways. Q: When it comes to preventing cardiovascular diseases, what are some key steps that people can take? A: One of the most important steps is to maintain a healthy lifestyle, including regular exercise, a balanced diet, and not smoking. It's also important to manage any underlying health conditions, such as high blood pressure and diabetes. Regular check-ups with a healthcare provider can also help identify any potential issues before they become more serious. Q: What advice would you give to someone who has recently been diagnosed with a cardiovascular disease? A: It's important to be proactive and take an active role in managing your condition. This includes following any prescribed treatments or medications, making lifestyle changes, and attending regular check-ups with your healthcare provider. It's also important to seek emotional and psychological support, as dealing with a cardiovascular disease can be a stressful and challenging experience. In conclusion, speaking with a cardiologist can provide valuable insights into the field of cardiology and the management of cardiovascular diseases. By taking steps to maintain a healthy lifestyle and be proactive in seeking care, individuals can reduce their risk of developing these conditions and lead fulfilling lives.